The Ultimate W: Busy People

Do Not Miss these Amazing Recipes to Lose Weight and Have Delicious Meals

Crystal Figueroa

Table of contents

Chipotle Chili Pork Chops

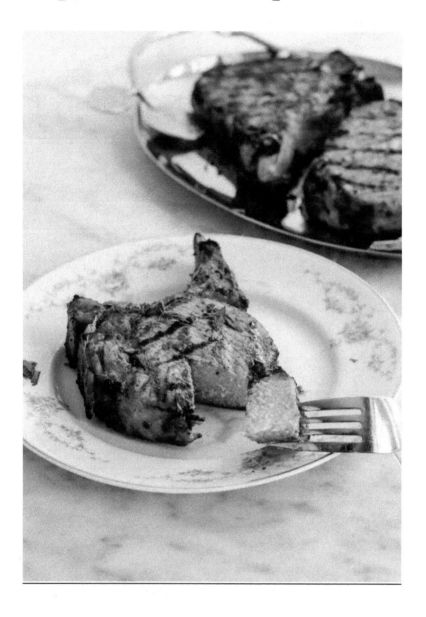

Preparation Time : 4 hours

Cooking Time : 20 minutes

Serving : 4

Ingredients :

- Juice and zest of 1 lime
- 1 tablespoon extra-virgin olive oil
- 1 tablespoon chipotle chili powder
- 2 teaspoons minced garlic
- 1 teaspoon ground cinnamon
- Pinch sea salt
- 4 (5-ounce) pork chops

Directions :

1. Combine the lime juice and zest, oil, chipotle chili powder, garlic, cinnamon, and salt in a resealable plastic bag. Add the pork chops. Remove as much air as possible and seal the bag.

2. Marinate the chops in the refrigerator for at least 4 hours, and up to 24 hours, turning them several times.

3. Ready the oven to 400°F and set a rack on a baking sheet. Let the chops rest at room temperature for 15 minutes, then arrange them on the rack and discard the remaining marinade.

4. Roast the chops until cooked through, turning once, about 10 minutes per side.

5. Serve with lime wedges.

Nutrition: 204 Calories; 1g Carbohydrates; 1g Sugar

Orange-Marinated Pork Tenderloin

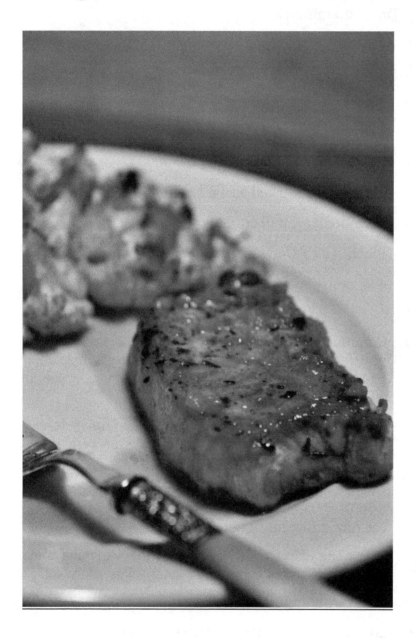

Preparation Time : 2 hours

Cooking Time : 30 minutes

Serving : 4

Ingredients :

- ¼ cup freshly squeezed orange juice

- 2 teaspoons orange zest

- 2 teaspoons minced garlic

- 1 teaspoon low-sodium soy sauce

- 1 teaspoon grated fresh ginger

- 1 teaspoon honey

- 1½ pounds pork tenderloin roast

- 1 tablespoon extra-virgin olive oil

Directions :

1. Blend together the orange juice, zest, garlic, soy sauce, ginger, and honey.

2. Pour the marinade into a resealable plastic bag and add the pork tenderloin.

3. Remove as much air as possible and seal the bag. Marinate the pork in the refrigerator, turning the bag a few times, for 2 hours.

4. Preheat the oven to 400°F.

5. Pull out tenderloin from the marinade and discard the marinade.

6. Position big ovenproof skillet over medium-high heat and add the oil.

7. Sear the pork tenderloin on all sides, about 5 minutes in total.

8. Position skillet to the oven and roast for 25 minutes.

9. Put aside for 10 minutes before serving.

Nutrition : 228 Calories; 4g Carbohydrates; 3g Sugar

Homestyle Herb Meatballs

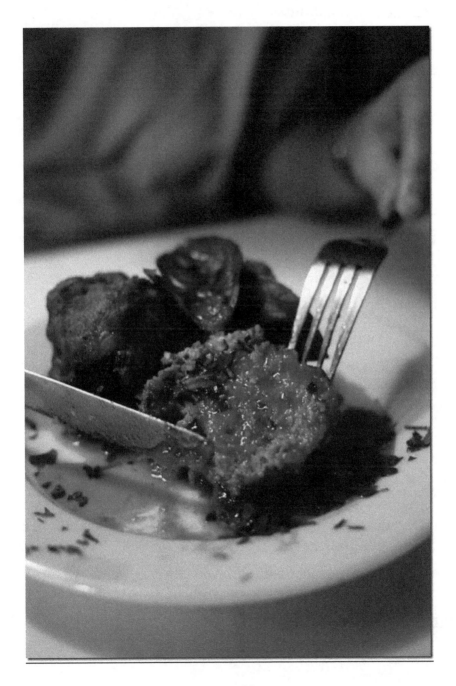

Preparation Time : 10 minutes

Cooking Time : 15 minutes

Serving : 4

Ingredients :

- ½ pound lean ground pork
- ½ pound lean ground beef
- 1 sweet onion, finely chopped
- ¼ cup bread crumbs
- 2 tablespoons chopped fresh basil
- 2 teaspoons minced garlic
- 1 egg

Directions :

1. Preheat the oven to 350°F.
2. Ready baking tray with parchment paper and set it aside.
3. In a large bowl, mix together the pork, beef, onion, bread crumbs, basil, garlic, egg, salt, and pepper until very well mixed.
4. Roll the meat mixture into 2-inch meatballs.
5. Transfer the meatballs to the baking sheet and bake until they are browned and cooked through, about 15 minutes.
6. Serve the meatballs with your favorite marinara sauce and some steamed green beans.

Nutrition : 332 Calories; 13g Carbohydrates; 3g Sugar

Lime-Parsley Lamb Cutlets

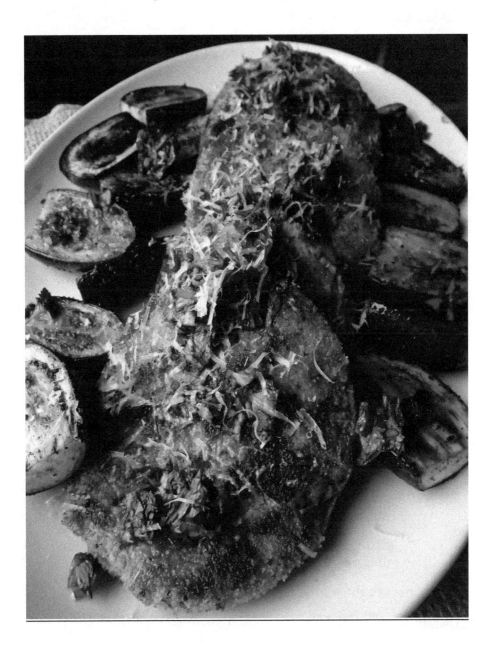

Preparation Time : 4 hours

Cooking Time : 10 minutes

Serving : 4

Ingredients :

- ¼ cup extra-virgin olive oil
- ¼ cup freshly squeezed lime juice
- 2 tablespoons lime zest
- 2 tablespoons chopped fresh parsley
- 12 lamb cutlets (about 1½ pounds total)

Directions :

1. Scourge the oil, lime juice, zest, parsley, salt, and pepper.
2. Pour marinade to a resealable plastic bag.
3. Add the cutlets to the bag and remove as much air as possible before sealing.
4. Marinate the lamb in the refrigerator for about 4 hours, turning the bag several times.
5. Preheat the oven to broil.
6. Remove the chops from the bag and arrange them on an aluminum foil–lined baking sheet. Discard the marinade.
7. Broil the chops for 4 minutes per side for medium doneness.
8. Let the chops rest for 5 minutes before serving.

Nutrition : 413 Calories; 1g Carbohydrates; 31g Protein

Mediterranean Steak Sandwiches

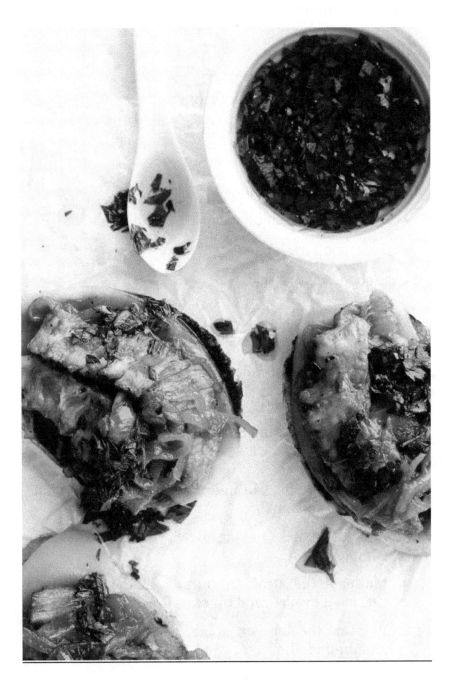

Preparation Time : 1 hour

Cooking Time : 10 minutes

Serving : 4

Ingredients :

- 2 tablespoons extra-virgin olive oil
- 2 tablespoons balsamic vinegar
- 2 teaspoons garlic
- 2 teaspoons lemon juice
- 2 teaspoons fresh oregano
- 1 teaspoon fresh parsley
- 1-pound flank steak
- 4 whole-wheat pitas
- 2 cups shredded lettuce
- 1 red onion, thinly sliced
- 1 tomato, chopped
- 1 ounce low-sodium feta cheese

Directions :

1. Scourge olive oil, balsamic vinegar, garlic, lemon juice, oregano, and parsley.
2. Add the steak to the bowl, turning to coat it completely.
3. Marinate the steak for 1 hour in the refrigerator, turning it over several times.
4. Preheat the broiler. Line a baking sheet with aluminum foil.

5. Put steak out of the bowl and discard the marinade.

6. Situate steak on the baking sheet and broil for 5 minutes per side for medium.

7. Set aside for 10 minutes before slicing.

8. Stuff the pitas with the sliced steak, lettuce, onion, tomato, and feta.

Nutrition : 344 Calories; 22g Carbohydrates; 3g Fiber

Roasted Beef with Peppercorn Sauce

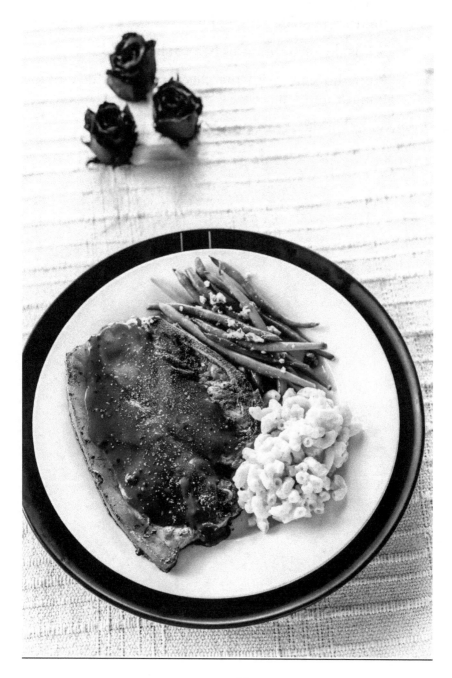

Preparation Time : 10 minutes

Cooking Time : 90 minutes

Serving : 4

Ingredients :

- 1½ pounds top rump beef roast
- 3 teaspoons extra-virgin olive oil
- 3 shallots, minced
- 2 teaspoons minced garlic
- 1 tablespoon green peppercorns
- 2 tablespoons dry sherry
- 2 tablespoons all-purpose flour
- 1 cup sodium-free beef broth

Directions :

1. Heat the oven to 300°F.
2. Season the roast with salt and pepper.
3. Position huge skillet over medium-high heat and add 2 teaspoons of olive oil.
4. Brown the beef on all sides, about 10 minutes in total, and transfer the roast to a baking dish.
5. Roast until desired doneness, about 1½ hours for medium. When the roast has been in the oven for 1 hour, start the sauce.
6. In a medium saucepan over medium-high heat, sauté the shallots in the remaining 1 teaspoon of olive oil until translucent, about 4 minutes.

7. Stir in the garlic and peppercorns, and cook for another minute. Whisk in the sherry to deglaze the pan.

8. Whisk in the flour to form a thick paste, cooking for 1 minute and stirring constantly.

9. Fill in the beef broth and whisk for 4 minutes. Season the sauce.

10. Serve the beef with a generous spoonful of sauce.

Nutrition : 330 Calories; 4g Carbohydrates; 36g Protein

Coffee-and-Herb-Marinated Steak

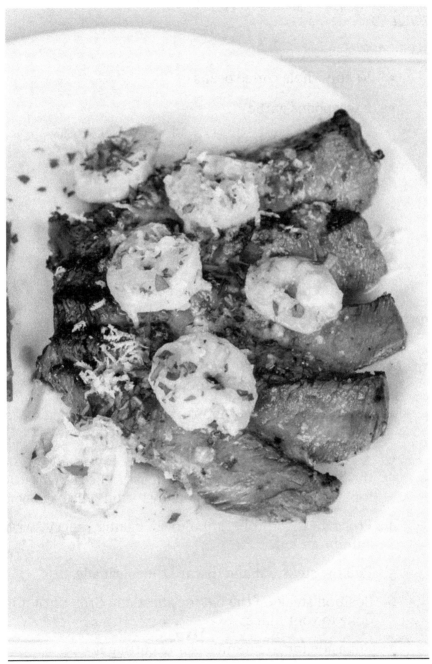

Preparation Time : 2 hours

Cooking Time : 10 minutes

Serving : 3

Ingredients :

- ¼ cup whole coffee beans
- 2 teaspoons garlic
- 2 teaspoons rosemary
- 2 teaspoons thyme
- 1 teaspoon black pepper
- 2 tablespoons apple cider vinegar
- 2 tablespoons extra-virgin olive oil
- 1-pound flank steak, trimmed of visible fat

Directions :

1. Place the coffee beans, garlic, rosemary, thyme, and black pepper in a coffee grinder or food processor and pulse until coarsely ground.

2. Transfer the coffee mixture to a resealable plastic bag and add the vinegar and oil. Shake to combine.

3. Add the flank steak and squeeze the excess air out of the bag. Seal it. Marinate the steak in the refrigerator for at least 2 hours, occasionally turning the bag over.

4. Preheat the broiler. Line a baking sheet with aluminum foil.

5. Pull the steak out and discard the marinade.

6. Position steak on the baking sheet and broil until it is done to your liking.

7. Put aside for 10 minutes before cutting it.

8. Serve with your favorite side dish.

Nutrition : 313 Calories; 20g Fat; 31g Protein

Traditional Beef Stroganoff

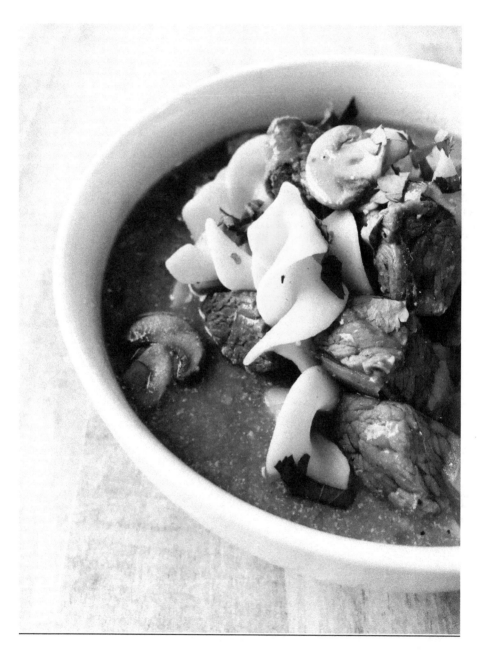

Preparation Time : 10 minutes

Cooking Time : 30 minutes

Serving : 4

Ingredients :

- 1 teaspoon extra-virgin olive oil
- 1-pound top sirloin, cut into thin strips
- 1 cup sliced button mushrooms
- ½ sweet onion, finely chopped
- 1 teaspoon minced garlic
- 1 tablespoon whole-wheat flour
- ½ cup low-sodium beef broth
- ¼ cup dry sherry
- ½ cup fat-free sour cream
- 1 tablespoon chopped fresh parsley

Direction :

1. Position the skillet over medium-high heat and add the oil.

2. Sauté the beef until browned, about 10 minutes, then remove the beef with a slotted spoon to a plate and set it aside.

3. Add the mushrooms, onion, and garlic to the skillet and sauté until lightly browned, about 5 minutes.

4. Whisk in the flour and then whisk in the beef broth and sherry.

5. Return the sirloin to the skillet and bring the mixture to a boil.

6. Reduce the heat to low and simmer until the beef is tender, about 10 minutes.

7. Stir in the sour cream and parsley. Season with salt and pepper.

Nutrition : 257 Calories; 6g Carbohydrates; 1g Fiber

Chicken and Roasted Vegetable Wraps

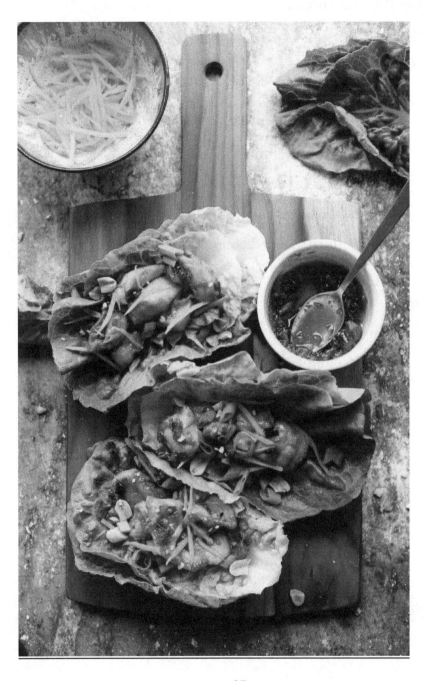

Preparation Time : 10 minutes

Cooking Time : 20 minutes

Serving : 4

Ingredients :

- ½ small eggplant
- 1 red bell pepper
- 1 medium zucchini
- ½ small red onion, sliced
- 1 tablespoon extra-virgin olive oil
- 2 (8-ounce) cooked chicken breasts, sliced
- 4 whole-wheat tortilla wraps

Directions :

1. Preheat the oven to 400°F.
2. Wrap baking sheet with foil and set it aside.
3. In a large bowl, toss the eggplant, bell pepper, zucchini, and red onion with the olive oil.
4. Transfer the vegetables to the baking sheet and lightly season with salt and pepper.
5. Roast the vegetables until soft and slightly charred, about 20 minutes.
6. Divide the vegetables and chicken into four portions.
7. Wrap 1 tortilla around each portion of chicken and grilled vegetables, and serve.

Nutrition : 483 Calories; 45g Carbohydrates; 3g Fiber

Ground Turkey Salad

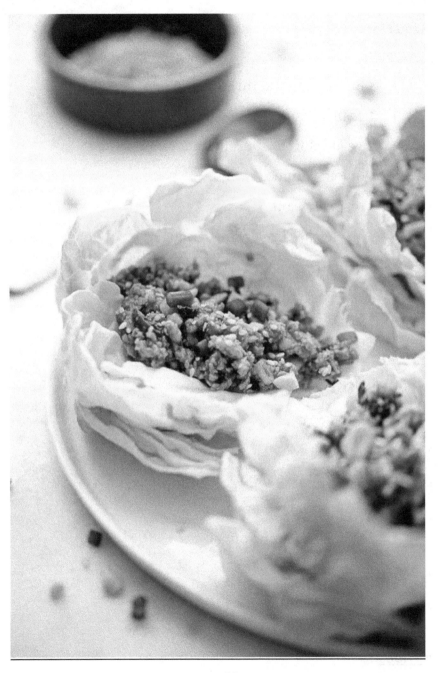

Preparation Time : 10 minutes

Cooking Time : 35 minutes

Servings : 6

Ingredients :

- 1 lb. lean ground turkey
- 1/2-inch ginger, minced
- 2 garlic cloves, minced
- 1 onion, chopped
- 1 tbsp. olive oil
- 1 bag lettuce leaves (for serving)
- ¼ cup fresh cilantro, chopped
- 2 tsp. coriander powder
- 1 tsp. red chili powder
- 1 tsp. turmeric powder
- Salt to taste
- 4 cups water

Dressing:

- 2 tbsp. fat free yogurt
- 1 tbsp. sour cream, non-fat
- 1 tbsp. low fat mayonnaise
- 1 lemon, juiced
- 1 tsp. red chili flakes
- Salt and pepper to taste

Directions :

1. In a skillet sauté the garlic and ginger in olive oil for 1 minute. Add onion and season with salt. Cook for 10 minutes over medium heat.

2. Add the ground turkey and sauté for 3 more minutes. Add the spices (turmeric, red chili powder and coriander powder).

3. Add 4 cups water and cook for 30 minutes, covered.

4. Prepare the dressing by combining yogurt, sour cream, mayo, lemon juice, chili flakes, salt and pepper.

5. To serve arrange the salad leaves on serving plates and place the cooked ground turkey on them. Top with dressing.

Nutrition : Carbohydrates: 9.1 g; Protein: 17.8 g; Total sugars: 2.5 g; Calories: 176

Asian Cucumber Salad

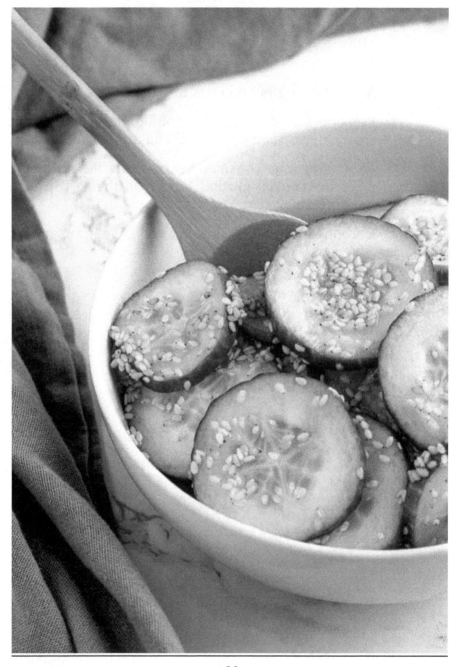

Preparation Time : 10 minutes

Cooking Time : none

Servings : 6

Ingredients :

- 1 lb. cucumbers, sliced
- 2 scallions, sliced
- 2 tbsp. sliced pickled ginger, chopped
- ¼ cup cilantro
- 1/2 red jalapeño, chopped
- 3 tbsp. rice wine vinegar
- 1 tbsp. sesame oil
- 1 tbsp. sesame seeds

Directions :

1. In a salad bowl combine all ingredients and toss together.

Nutrition : Carbohydrates: 5.7 g; Protein: 1 g; Total sugars: 3.1 g; Calories: 52

Cauliflower Tofu Salad

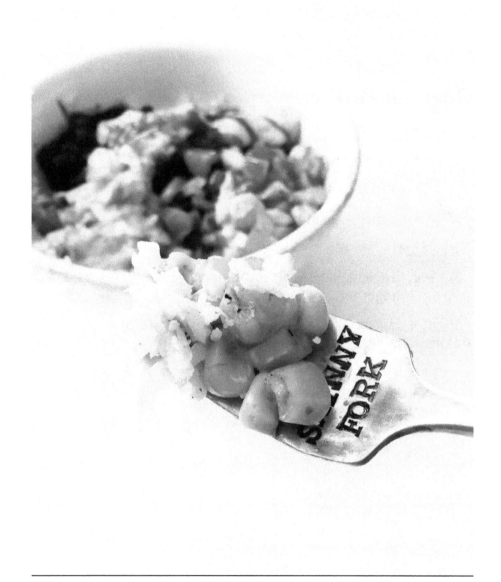

Preparation Time : 10 minutes

Cooking Time : 15 minutes

Servings : 4

Ingredients :

- 2 cups cauliflower florets, blended
- 1 fresh cucumber, diced
- 1/2 cup green olives, diced
- 1/3 cup red onion, diced
- 2 tbsp. toasted pine nuts
- 2 tbsp. raisins
- 1/3 cup feta, crumbled
- 1/2 cup pomegranate seeds
- 2 lemons (juiced, zest grated)
- 8 oz. tofu
- 2 tsp. oregano
- 2 garlic cloves, minced
- 1/2 tsp. red chili flakes
- 3 tbsp. olive oil
- Salt and pepper to taste

Directions :

1. Season the processed cauliflower with salt and transfer to a strainer to drain.

2. Prepare the marinade for tofu by combining 2 tbsp. lemon juice, 1.5 tbsp. olive oil, minced garlic, chili

flakes, oregano, salt and pepper. Coat tofu in the marinade and set aside.

3. Preheat the oven to 450F.

4. Bake tofu on a baking sheet for 12 minutes.

5. In a salad bowl mix the remaining marinade with onions, cucumber, cauliflower, olives and raisins. Add in the remaining olive oil and grated lemon zest.

6. Top with tofu, pine nuts, and feta and pomegranate seeds.

Nutrition : Carbohydrates: 34.1 g; Protein: 11.1 g; Total sugars: 11.5 g; Calories: 328

Scallop Caesar Salad

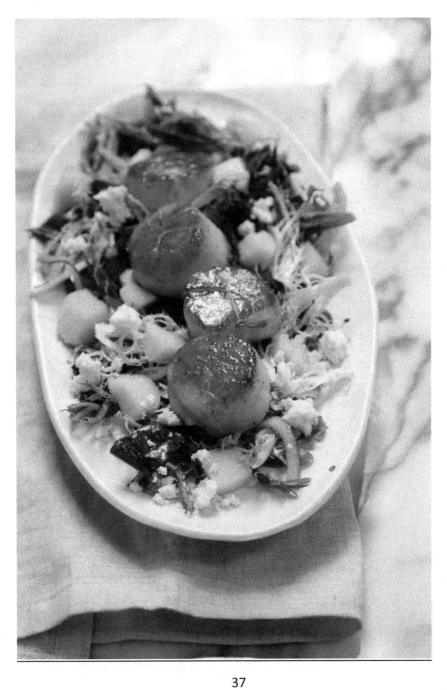

Preparation Time : 5 minutes

Cooking Time : 2 minutes

Servings : 2

Ingredients :

- 8 sea scallops
- 4 cups romaine lettuce
- 2 tsp. olive oil
- 3 tbsp. Caesar Salad Dressing
- 1 tsp. lemon juice
- Salt and pepper to taste

Directions:

1. In a frying pan heat olive oil and cook the scallops in one layer no longer than 2 minutes per both sides. Season with salt and pepper to taste.

2. Arrange lettuce on plates and place scallops on top.

3. Pour over the Caesar dressing and lemon juice.

Nutrition : Carbohydrates: 14 g; Protein: 30.7 g; Total sugars: 2.2 g; Calories: 340 g

Chicken Avocado Salad

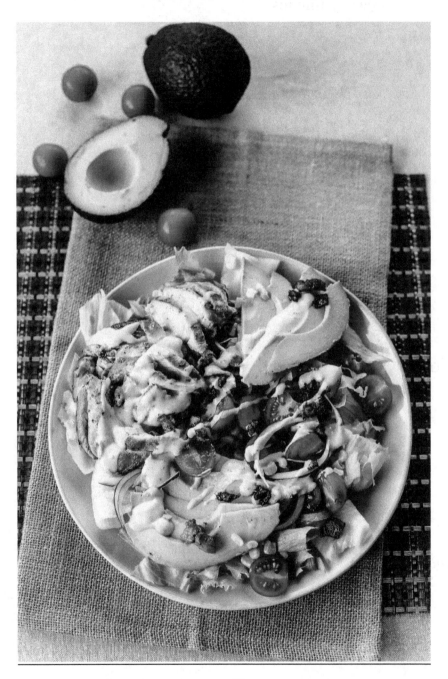

Preparation Time : 30 minutes

Cooking Time : 15 minutes

Servings : 4

Ingredients :

- 1 lb. chicken breast, cooked, shredded
- 1 avocado, pitted, peeled, sliced
- 2 tomatoes, diced
- 1 cucumber, peeled, sliced
- 1 head lettuce, chopped
- 3 tbsp. olive oil
- 2 tbsp. lime juice
- 1 tbsp. cilantro, chopped
- Salt and pepper to taste

Directions :

1. In a bowl whisk together oil, lime juice, cilantro, salt, and a pinch of pepper.
2. Combine lettuce, tomatoes, cucumber in a salad bowl and toss with half of the dressing.
3. Toss chicken with the remaining dressing and combine with vegetable mixture.
4. Top with avocado.

Nutrition : Carbohydrates: 10 g; Protein: 38 g; Total sugars: 11.5 g; Calories: 380

California Wraps

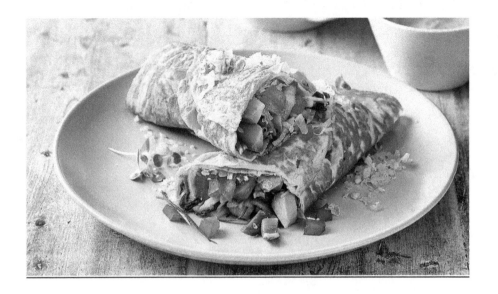

Preparation Time : 5 minutes

Cooking Time : 15 minutes

Servings : 4

Ingredients :

- 4 slices turkey breast, cooked
- 4 slices ham, cooked
- 4 lettuce leaves
- 4 slices tomato
- 4 slices avocado
- 1 tsp. lime juice
- A handful watercress leaves
- 4 tbsp. Ranch dressing, sugar free

Directions :

1. Top a lettuce leaf with turkey slice, ham slice and tomato.

2. In a bowl combine avocado and lime juice and place on top of tomatoes. Top with water cress and dressing.

3. Repeat with the remaining ingredients for 4. Topping each lettuce leaf with a turkey slice, ham slice, tomato and dressing.

Nutrition : Carbohydrates: 4 g; Protein: 9 g; Total sugars: 0.5 g; Calories: 140

Chicken Salad in Cucumber Cups

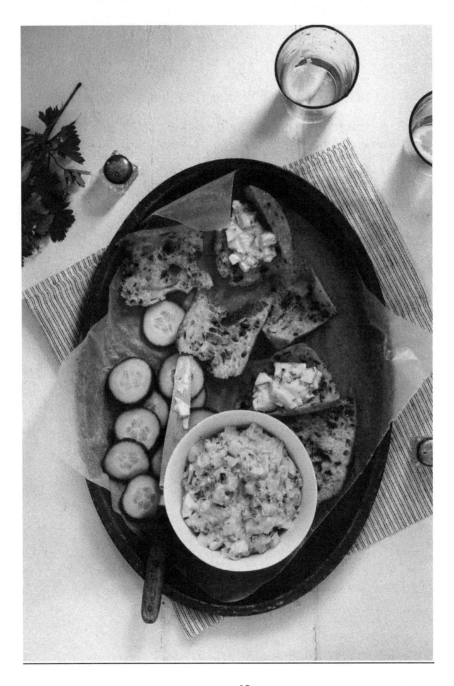

Preparation Time : 5 minutes

Cooking Time : 15 minutes

Servings : 4

Ingredients :

- 1/2 chicken breast, skinless, boiled and shredded
- 2 long cucumbers, cut into 8 thick rounds each, scooped out (won't use in a).
- 1 tsp. ginger, minced
- 1 tsp. lime zest, grated
- 4 tsp. olive oil
- 1 tsp. sesame oil
- 1 tsp. lime juice
- Salt and pepper to taste

Directions :

1. In a bowl combine lime zest, juice, olive and sesame oils, ginger, and season with salt.
2. Toss the chicken with the dressing and fill the cucumber cups with the salad.

Nutrition : Carbohydrates: 4 g; Protein: 12 g; Total sugars: 0.5 g; Calories: 116 g

Sunflower Seeds and Arugula Garden Salad

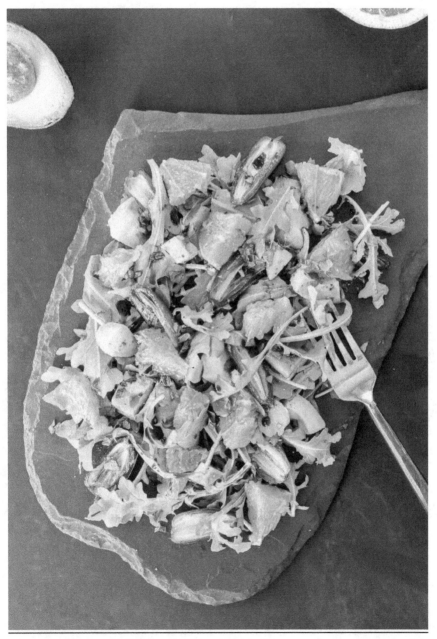

Preparation Time : 5 minutes

Cooking Time : 10 minutes

Servings : 6

Ingredients :

- ¼ tsp. black pepper
- ¼ tsp. salt
- 1 tsp. fresh thyme, chopped
- 2 tbsp. sunflower seeds, toasted
- 2 cups red grapes, halved
- 7 cups baby arugula, loosely packed
- 1 tbsp. coconut oil
- 2 tsp. honey
- 3 tbsp. red wine vinegar
- 1/2 tsp. stone-ground mustard

Directions :

1. In a small bowl, whisk together mustard, honey and vinegar. Slowly pour oil as you whisk.

2. In a large salad bowl, mix thyme, seeds, grapes and arugula.

3. Drizzle with dressing and serve.

Nutrition : Calories: 86.7g; Protein: 1.6g; Carbs: 13.1g; Fat: 3.1g

Supreme Caesar Salad

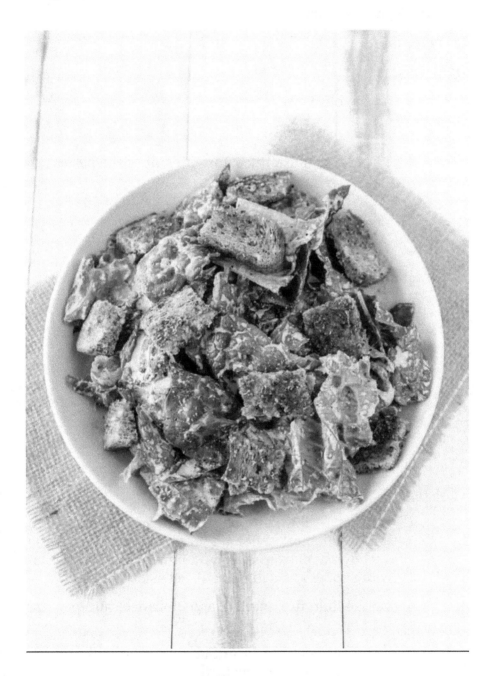

Preparation Time : 5 minutes

Cooking Time : 10 minutes

Servings : 4

Ingredients :

- ¼ cup olive oil
- ¾ cup mayonnaise
- 1 head romaine lettuce, torn into bite sized pieces
- 1 tbsp. lemon juice
- 1 tsp. Dijon mustard
- 1 tsp. Worcestershire sauce
- 3 cloves garlic, peeled and minced
- 3 cloves garlic, peeled and quartered
- 4 cups day old bread, cubed
- 5 anchovy filets, minced
- 6 tbsp. grated parmesan cheese, divided
- Ground black pepper to taste
- Salt to taste

Directions :

1. In a small bowl, whisk well lemon juice, mustard, Worcestershire sauce, 2 tbsp. parmesan cheese, anchovies, mayonnaise, and minced garlic. Season with pepper and salt to taste. Set aside in the ref.

2. On medium fire, place a large nonstick saucepan and heat oil.

3. Sauté quartered garlic until browned around a minute or two. Remove and discard.

4. Add bread cubes in same pan, sauté until lightly browned. Season with pepper and salt. Transfer to a plate.

5. In large bowl, place lettuce and pour in dressing. Toss well to coat. Top with remaining parmesan cheese.

6. Garnish with bread cubes, serve, and enjoy.

Nutrition : Calories: 443.3g; Fat: 32.1g; Protein: 11.6g; Carbs: 27g

Tabbouleh- Arabian Salad

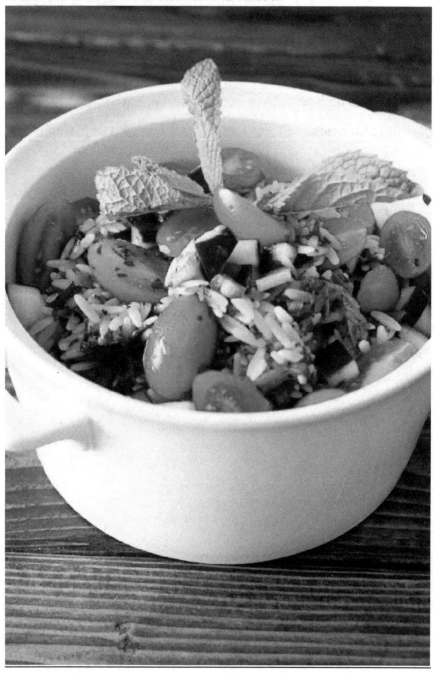

Preparation Time : 5 minutes

Cooking Time : 10 minutes

Servings : 6

Ingredients :

- ¼ cup chopped fresh mint
- 1 2/3 cups boiling water
- 1 cucumber, peeled, seeded and chopped
- 1 cup bulgur
- 1 cup chopped fresh parsley
- 1 cup chopped green onions
- 1 tsp. salt
- 1/3 cup lemon juice
- 1/3 cup olive oil
- 3 tomatoes, chopped
- Ground black pepper to taste

Directions :

1. In a large bowl, mix together boiling water and bulgur. Let soak and set aside for an hour while covered.

2. After one hour, toss in cucumber, tomatoes, mint, parsley, onions, lemon juice and oil. Then season with black pepper and salt to taste. Toss well and refrigerate for another hour while covered before serving.

Nutrition : Calories: 185.5g; Fat: 13.1g; Protein: 4.1g; Carbs: 12.8g

Aromatic Toasted Pumpkin Seeds

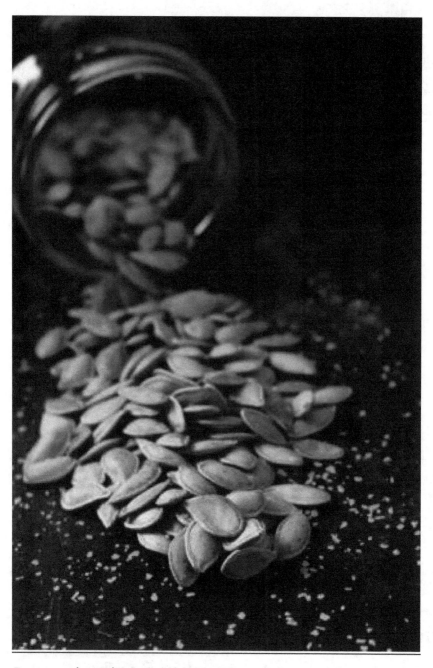

Preparation Time : 5 minutes

Cooking Time : 45 minutes

Serving : 4

Ingredients :

- 1 cup pumpkin seeds

- 1 teaspoon cinnamon

- 2 packets stevia

- 1 tablespoon canola oil

- ¼ teaspoon sea salt

Directions :

1. Prep the oven to 300°F (150°C).

2. Combine the pumpkin seeds with cinnamon, stevia, canola oil, and salt in a bowl. Stir to mix well.

3. Pour the seeds in the single layer on a baking sheet, then arrange the sheet in the preheated oven.

4. Bake for 45 minutes or until well toasted and fragrant. Shake the sheet twice to bake the seeds evenly.

5. Serve immediately.

Nutrition : 202 Calories; 5.1g Carbohydrates; 2.3g Fiber

Bacon-Wrapped Shrimps

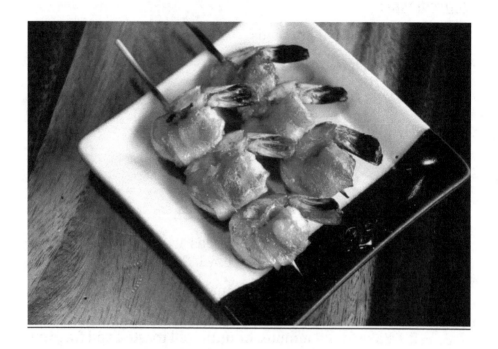

Preparation Time : 10 minutes

Cooking Time : 6 minutes

Serving : 10

Ingredients :

- 20 shrimps, peeled and deveined
- 7 slices bacon
- 4 leaves romaine lettuce

Directions :

1. Set the oven to 205°C.
2. Wrap each shrimp with each bacon strip, then arrange the wrapped shrimps in a single layer on a baking sheet, seam side down.
3. Broil for 6 minutes. Flip the shrimps halfway through the cooking time.
4. Take out from the oven and serve on lettuce leaves.

Nutrition : 70 Calories; 4.5g Fat; 7g Protein

Blackened Shrimp

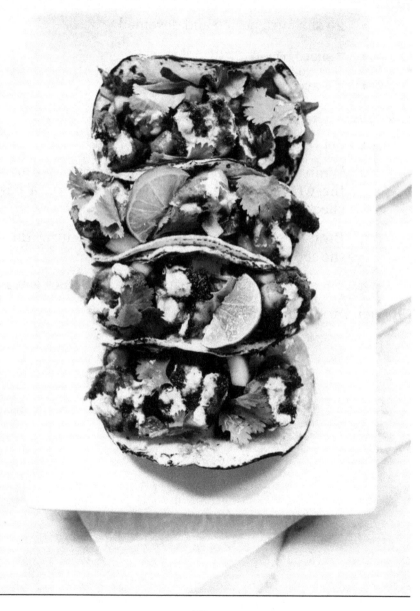

Preparation Time : 5 minutes

Cooking Time : 5 minutes

Servings : 4

Ingredients :

- 1 1/2 lbs. shrimp, peel & devein
- 4 lime wedges
- 4 tbsp. cilantro, chopped
- What you'll need from store cupboard:
- 4 cloves garlic, diced
- 1 tbsp. chili powder
- 1 tbsp. paprika
- 1 tbsp. olive oil
- 2 tsp. Splenda brown sugar
- 1 tsp. cumin
- 1 tsp. oregano
- 1 tsp. garlic powder
- 1 tsp. salt
- 1/2 tsp. pepper

Directions :

1. In a small bowl combine seasonings and Splenda brown sugar.

2. Heat oil in a skillet over med-high heat. Add shrimp, in a single layer, and cook 1-2 minutes per side.

3. Add seasonings, and cook, stirring, 30 seconds. Serve garnished with cilantro and a lime wedge.

<u>*Nutrition*</u> : Calories 252; Total Carbs 7g; Net Carbs 6g; Protein 39g; Fat 7g; Sugar 2g; Fiber 1g

Cajun Catfish

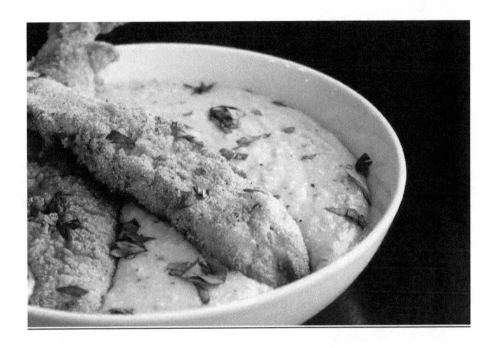

Preparation Time : 5 minutes

Cooking Time : 15 minutes

Servings : 4

Ingredients :

- 4 (8 oz.) catfish fillets
- What you'll need from store cupboard:
- 2 tbsp. olive oil
- 2 tsp. garlic salt
- 2 tsp. thyme
- 2 tsp. paprika
- 1/2 tsp. cayenne pepper
- 1/2 tsp. red hot sauce
- ¼ tsp. black pepper
- Nonstick cooking spray

Directions :

1. Heat oven to 450 degrees. Spray a 9x13-inch baking dish with cooking spray.

2. In a small bowl whisk together everything but catfish. Brush both sides of fillets, using all the spice mix.

3. Bake 10-13 minutes or until fish flakes easily with a fork. Serve.

Nutrition : Calories 366; Total Carbs 0g; Protein 35g; Fat 24g; Sugar 0g; Fiber 0g

Cajun Flounder & Tomatoes

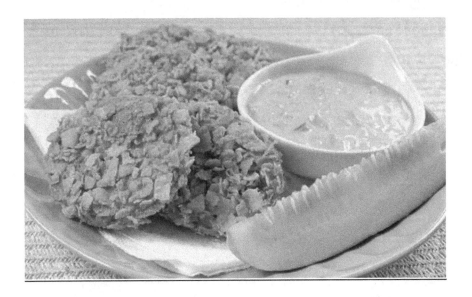

Preparation Time : 10 minutes

Cooking Time : 15 minutes

Servings : 4

Ingredients :

- 4 flounder fillets
- 2 1/2 cups tomatoes, diced
- ¾ cup onion, diced
- ¾ cup green bell pepper, diced
- What you'll need from store cupboard:
- 2 cloves garlic, diced fine
- 1 tbsp. Cajun seasoning
- 1 tsp. olive oil

Directions :

1. Heat oil in a large skillet over med-high heat. Add onion and garlic and cook 2 minutes, or until soft. Add tomatoes, peppers and spices, and cook 2-3 minutes until tomatoes soften.

2. Lay fish over top. Cover, reduce heat to medium and cook, 5-8 minutes, or until fish flakes easily with a fork. Transfer fish to serving plates and top with sauce.

Nutrition : Calories 194; Total Carbs 8g; Net Carbs 6g; Protein 32g; Fat 3g; Sugar 5g; Fiber 2g

Cajun Shrimp & Roasted Vegetables

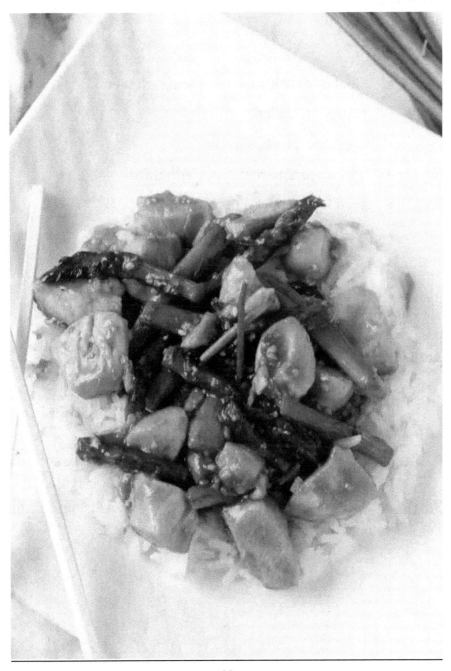

Preparation Time : 5 minutes

Cooking Time : 15 minutes

Servings : 4

Ingredients :

- 1 lb. large shrimp, peeled and deveined

- 2 zucchinis, sliced

- 2 yellow squash, sliced

- 1/2 bunch asparagus, cut into thirds

- 2 red bell pepper, cut into chunks

- What you'll need from store cupboard:

- 2 tbsp. olive oil

- 2 tbsp. Cajun Seasoning

- Salt & pepper, to taste

Directions :

1. Heat oven to 400 degrees.

2. Combine shrimp and vegetables in a large bowl. Add oil and seasoning and toss to coat.

3. Spread evenly in a large baking sheet and bake 15-20 minutes, or until vegetables are tender. Serve.

Nutrition : Calories 251; Total Carbs 13g; Net Carbs 9g; Protein 30g; Fat 9g; Sugar 6g; Fiber 4g

Cilantro Lime Grilled Shrimp

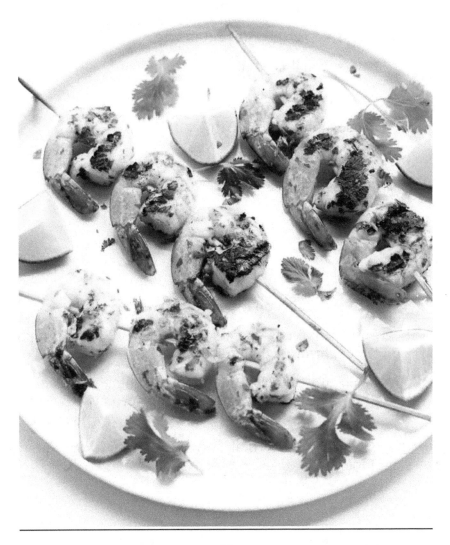

Preparation Time : 5 minutes

Cooking Time : 5 minutes

Servings : 6

Ingredients :

- 1 1/2 lbs. large shrimp raw, peeled, deveined with tails on
- Juice and zest of 1 lime
- 2 tbsp. fresh cilantro chopped
- What you'll need from store cupboard:
- ¼ cup olive oil
- 2 cloves garlic, diced fine
- 1 tsp. smoked paprika
- ¼ tsp. cumin
- 1/2 teaspoon salt
- ¼ tsp. cayenne pepper

Directions :

1. Place the shrimp in a large Ziploc bag.
2. Mix remaining Ingredients in a small bowl and pour over shrimp. Let marinate 20-30 minutes.
3. Heat up the grill. Skewer the shrimp and cook 2-3 minutes, per side, just until they turn pick. Be careful not to overcook them. Serve garnished with cilantro.

Nutrition : Calories 317; Total Carbs 4g; Protein 39g; Fat 15g; Sugar 0g; Fiber 0g

Crab Frittata

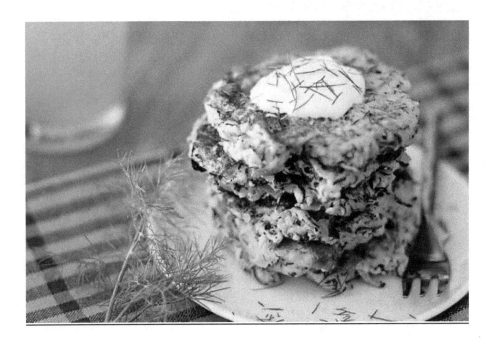

Preparation Time : 10 minutes

Cooking Time : 50 minutes

Servings : 4

Ingredients :

- 4 eggs
- 2 cups lump crabmeat
- 1 cup half-n-half
- 1 cup green onions, diced
- What you'll need from store cupboard:
- 1 cup reduced fat parmesan cheese, grated
- 1 tsp. salt
- 1 tsp. pepper
- 1 tsp. smoked paprika
- 1 tsp. Italian seasoning
- Nonstick cooking spray

Directions :

1. Heat oven to 350 degrees. Spray an 8-inch springform pan, or pie plate with cooking spray.

2. In a large bowl, whisk together the eggs and half-n-half. Add seasonings and parmesan cheese, stir to mix.

3. Stir in the onions and crab meat. Pour into prepared pan and bake 35-40 minutes, or eggs are set and top is lightly browned.

4. Let cool 10 minutes, then slice and serve warm or at room temperature.

Nutrition : Calories 276; Total Carbs 5g; Net Carbs 4g; Protein 25g; Fat 17g; Sugar 1g; Fiber 1g

Crunchy Lemon Shrimp

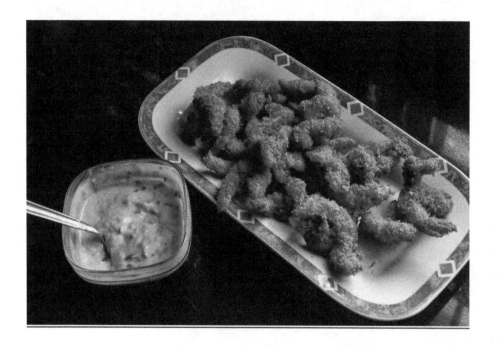

Preparation Time : 5 minutes

Cooking Time : 10 minutes

Servings : 4

Ingredients :

- 1 lb. raw shrimp, peeled and deveined
- 2 tbsp. Italian parsley, roughly chopped
- 2 tbsp. lemon juice, divided
- What you'll need from store cupboard:
- 2/3 cup panko bread crumbs
- 21/2 tbsp. olive oil, divided
- Salt and pepper, to taste

Directions :

1. Heat oven to 400 degrees.
2. Place the shrimp evenly in a baking dish and sprinkle with salt and pepper. Drizzle on 1 tablespoon lemon juice and 1 tablespoon of olive oil. Set aside.
3. In a medium bowl, combine parsley, remaining lemon juice, bread crumbs, remaining olive oil, and ¼ tsp. each of salt and pepper. Layer the panko mixture evenly on top of the shrimp.
4. Bake 8-10 minutes or until shrimp are cooked through and the panko is golden brown.

Nutrition : Calories 283; Total Carbs 15g; Net Carbs 14g; Protein 28g; Fat 12g; Sugar 1g; Fiber 1g

Grilled Tuna Steaks

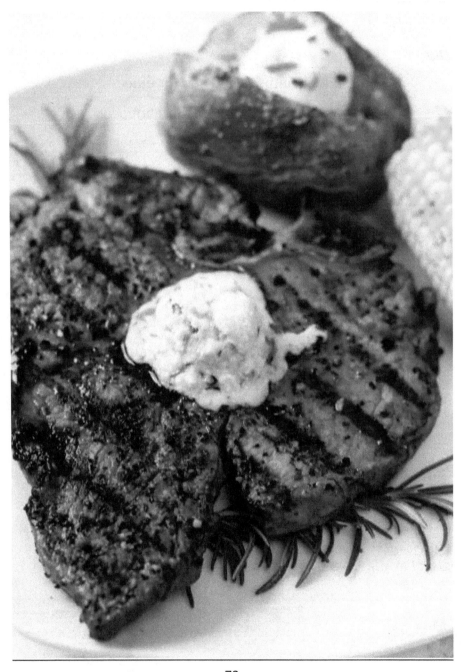

Preparation Time : 5 minutes

Cooking Time : 10 minutes

Servings : 6

Ingredients :

- 6 6 oz. tuna steaks
- 3 tbsp. fresh basil, diced
- What you'll need from store cupboard:
- 4 1/2 tsp. olive oil
- ¾ tsp. salt
- ¼ tsp. pepper
- Nonstick cooking spray

Directions :

1. Heat grill to medium heat. Spray rack with cooking spray.
2. Drizzle both sides of the tuna with oil. Sprinkle with basil, salt and pepper.
3. Place on grill and cook 5 minutes per side, tuna should be slightly pink in the center. Serve.

Nutrition : Calories 343; Total Carbs 0g; Protein 51g; Fat 14g; Sugar 0g; Fiber 0g

Red Clam Sauce & Pasta

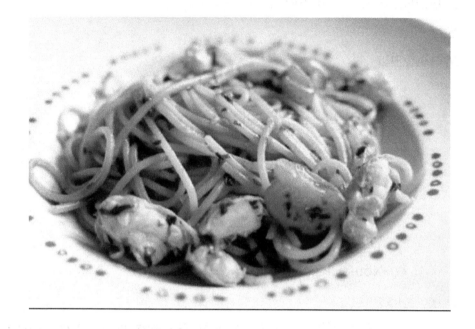

Preparation Time : 10 minutes

Cooking Time : 3 hours

Servings : 4

Ingredients :

- 1 onion, diced
- ¼ cup fresh parsley, diced
- What you'll need from store cupboard:
- 2 6 1/2 oz. cans clams, chopped, undrained
- 14 1/2 oz. tomatoes, diced, undrained
- 6 oz. tomato paste
- 2 cloves garlic, diced
- 1 bay leaf
- 1 tbsp. sunflower oil
- 1 tsp. Splenda
- 1 tsp. basil
- 1/2 tsp. thyme
- 1/2 Homemade Pasta, cook & drain

Directions :

1. Heat oil in a small skillet over med-high heat. Add onion and cook until tender, add garlic and cook 1 minute more. Transfer to crock pot.

2. Add remaining Ingredients, except pasta, cover and cook on low 3-4 hours.

3. Discard bay leaf and serve over cooked pasta.

Nutrition : Calories 223; Total Carbs 32g; Net Carbs 27g; Protein 12g; Fat 6g; Sugar 15g; Fiber 5g

Salmon Milano

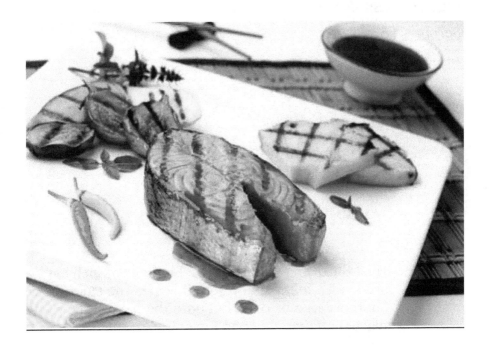

Preparation Time : 10 minutes

Cooking Time : 20 minutes

Servings : 6

Ingredients :

- 2 1/2 lb. salmon filet
- 2 tomatoes, sliced
- 1/2 cup margarine
- What you'll need from store cupboard:
- 1/2 cup basil pesto

Directions :

1. Heat the oven to 400 degrees. Line a 9x15-inch baking sheet with foil, making sure it covers the sides. Place another large piece of foil onto the baking sheet and place the salmon filet on top of it.

2. Place the pesto and margarine in blender or food processor and pulse until smooth. Spread evenly over salmon. Place tomato slices on top.

3. Wrap the foil around the salmon, tenting around the top to prevent foil from touching the salmon as much as possible. Bake 15-25 minutes, or salmon flakes easily with a fork. Serve.

Nutrition : Calories 444; Total Carbs 2g; Protein 55g; Fat 24g; Sugar 1g; Fiber 0g

Shrimp & Artichoke Skillet

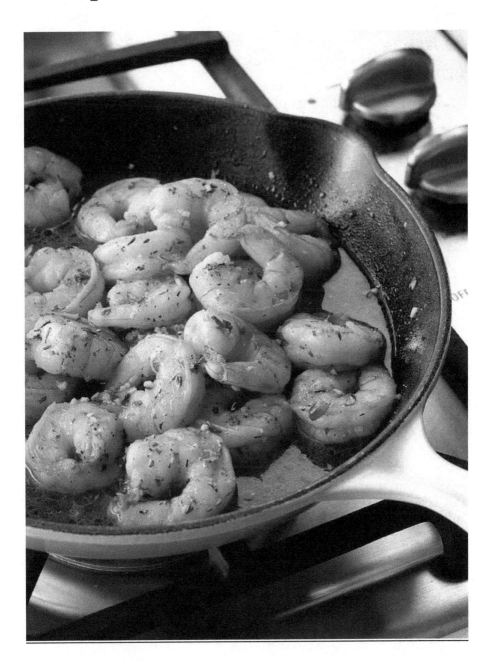

Preparation Time : 5 minutes

Cooking Time : 10 minutes

Servings : 4

Ingredients :

- 1 1/2 cups shrimp, peel & devein
- 2 shallots, diced
- 1 tbsp. margarine
- What you'll need from store cupboard
- 2 12 oz. jars artichoke hearts, drain & rinse
- 2 cups white wine
- 2 cloves garlic, diced fine

Directions :

1. Melt margarine in a large skillet over med-high heat. Add shallot and garlic and cook until they start to brown, stirring frequently.

2. Add artichokes and cook 5 minutes. Reduce heat and add wine. Cook 3 minutes, stirring occasionally.

3. Add the shrimp and cook just until they turn pink. Serve.

Nutrition : Calories 487; Total Carbs 26g; Net Carbs 17g; Protein 64g; Fat 5g; Sugar 3g; Fiber 9g

Tuna Carbonara

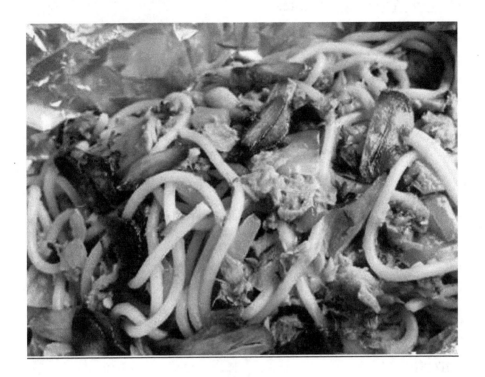

Preparation Time : 5 minutes

Cooking Time : 25 minutes

Servings : 4

Ingredients :

- 1/2 lb. tuna fillet, cut in pieces
- 2 eggs
- 4 tbsp. fresh parsley, diced
- What you'll need from store cupboard:
- 1/2 Homemade Pasta, cook & drain,
- 1/2 cup reduced fat parmesan cheese
- 2 cloves garlic, peeled
- 2 tbsp. extra virgin olive oil
- Salt & pepper, to taste

Directions :

1. In a small bowl, beat the eggs, parmesan and a dash of pepper.

2. Heat the oil in a large skillet over med-high heat. Add garlic and cook until browned. Add the tuna and cook 2-3 minutes, or until tuna is almost cooked through. Discard the garlic.

3. Add the pasta and reduce heat. Stir in egg mixture and cook, stirring constantly, 2 minutes. If the sauce is too thick, thin with water, a little bit at a time, until it has a creamy texture.

4. Salt and pepper to taste and serve garnished with parsley.

Nutrition : Calories 409; Total Carbs 7g; Net Carbs 6g; Protein 25g; Fat 30g; Sugar 3g; Fiber 1g

Mediterranean Fish Fillets

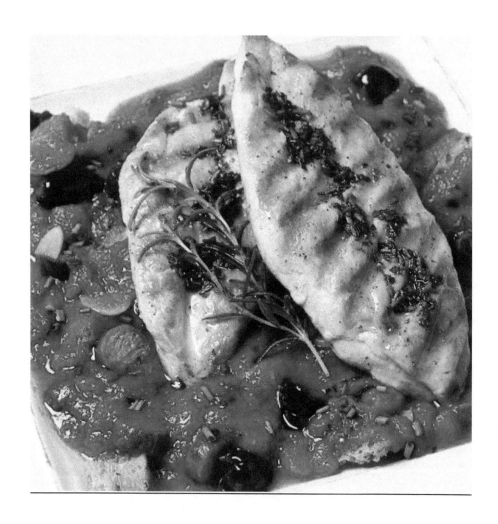

Preparation Time : 10 minutes

Cooking Time : 3 minutes

Servings : 4

Ingredients :

- 4 cod fillets
- 1 lb. grape tomatoes, halved
- 1 cup olives, pitted and sliced
- 2 tbsp. capers
- 1 tsp. dried thyme
- 2 tbsp. olive oil
- 1 tsp. garlic, minced
- Pepper
- Salt

Directions :

1. Pour 1 cup water into the Pressure Pot then place steamer rack in the pot.
2. Spray heat-safe baking dish with cooking spray.
3. Add half grape tomatoes into the dish and season with pepper and salt.
4. Arrange fish fillets on top of cherry tomatoes. Drizzle with oil and season with garlic, thyme, capers, pepper, and salt.
5. Spread olives and remaining grape tomatoes on top of fish fillets.
6. Place dish on top of steamer rack in the pot.

7. Seal pot with a lid and select manual and cook on high for 3 minutes.

8. Once done, release pressure using quick release. Remove lid.

9. Serve and enjoy.

Nutrition : Calories 212; Fat 11.9 g; Carbohydrates 7.1 g; Sugar 3 g; Protein 21.4 g; Cholesterol 55 mg

Cinnamon Cake

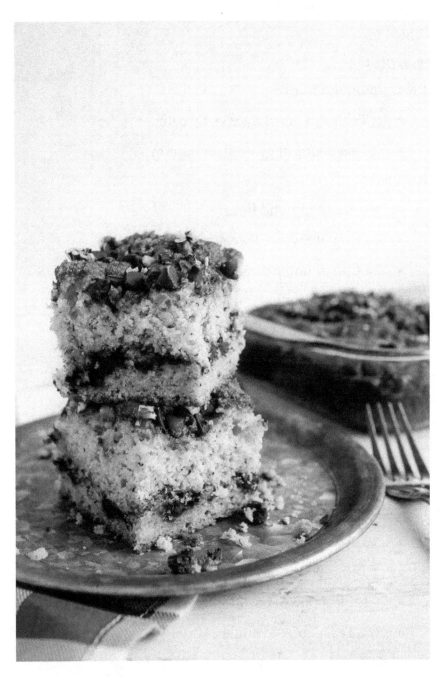

Preparation Time : 15 minutes

Cooking Time : 35minutes

Servings : 6

Ingredients :

For the Cinnamon Filling:

- 3 Tablespoons of Swerve Sweetener
- 2 Teaspoons of ground cinnamon

For the Cake:

- 3 Cups of almond flour
- ¾ Cup of Swerve Sweetener
- ¼ Cup of unflavored whey protein powder
- 2 Teaspoon of baking powder
- 1/2 Teaspoon of salt
- 3 large pastured eggs
- 1/2 Cup of melted coconut oil
- 1/2 Teaspoon of vanilla extract
- 1/2 Cup of almond milk
- 1 Tablespoon of melted coconut oil

For the cream cheese Frosting:

- 3 Tablespoons of softened cream cheese
- 2 Tablespoons of powdered Swerve Sweetener
- 1 Tablespoon of coconut heavy whipping cream
- 1/2 Teaspoon of vanilla extract

Directions:

1. Preheat your oven to a temperature of about 325 F and grease a baking tray of 8x8 inch.

2. For the filling, mix the Swerve and the cinnamon in a mixing bowl and mix very well; then set it aside.

3. For the preparation of the cake; whisk all together the almond flour, the sweetener, the protein powder, the baking powder, and the salt in a mixing bowl.

4. Add in the eggs, the melted coconut oil and the vanilla extract and mix very well.

5. Add in the almond milk and keep stirring until your ingredients are very well combined.

6. Spread about half of the batter in the prepared pan; then sprinkle with about two thirds of the filling mixture.

7. Spread the remaining mixture of the batter over the filling and smooth it with a spatula.

8. Bake for about 35 minutes in the oven.

9. Brush with the melted coconut oil and sprinkle with the remaining cinnamon filling.

10. Prepare the frosting by beating the cream cheese, the powdered erythritol, the cream and the vanilla extract in a mixing bowl until it becomes smooth.

11. Drizzle frost over the cooled cake.

12. Slice the cake; then serve and enjoy your cake!

Nutrition : Calories: 222; Fat: 19.2g; Carbohydrates: 5.4g; Fiber: 1.5g; Protein: 7.3g

Banana Nut Muffins

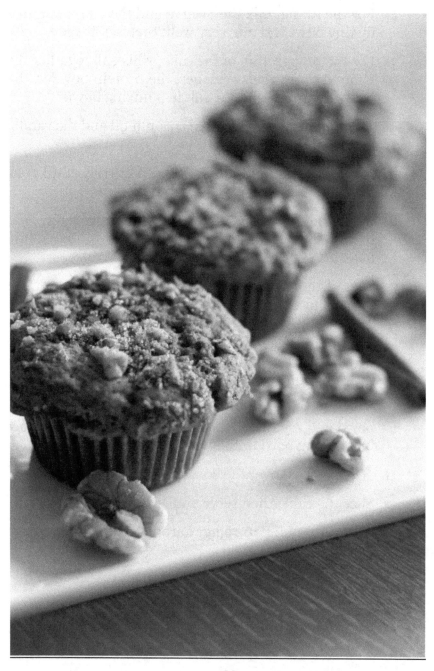

Preparation Time : 5 minutes

Cooking Time : 1 Hour

Servings : 6

Ingredients:

Dry Ingredients:

- 1 1/2 cups of Spell or Teff Flour
- 1/2 teaspoon of Pure Sea Salt
- 3/4 cup of Date Syrup

Wet Ingredients:

- 2 medium Blend Burro Bananas
- ¼ cup of Grape Seed Oil
- ¾ cup of Homemade Walnut Milk (see recipe)*
- 1 tablespoon of Key Lime Juice

Filling Ingredients:

- ½ cup of chopped Walnuts (plus extra for decorating)
- 1 chopped Burro Banana

Directions :

1. Preheat your oven to 400 degrees Fahrenheit.
2. Take a muffin tray and grease 12 cups or line with cupcake liners.
3. Put all dry Ingredients in a large bowl and mix them thoroughly.
4. Add all wet Ingredients to a separate, smaller bowl and mix well with Blend Bananas.

5. Mix Ingredients from the two bowls in one large container. Be careful not to over mix.

6. Add the filling Ingredients and fold in gently.

7. Pour muffin batter into the 12 prepared muffin cups and garnish with a couple Walnuts.

8. Bake it for 22 to 26 minutes until golden brown.

9. Allow to cool for 10 minutes.

10. Serve and enjoy your Banana Nut Muffins!

Nutrition : Calories: 150; Fat: 10 g; Carbohydrates: 30 g; Protein: 2.4 g; Fiber: 2 g

Mango Nut Cheesecake

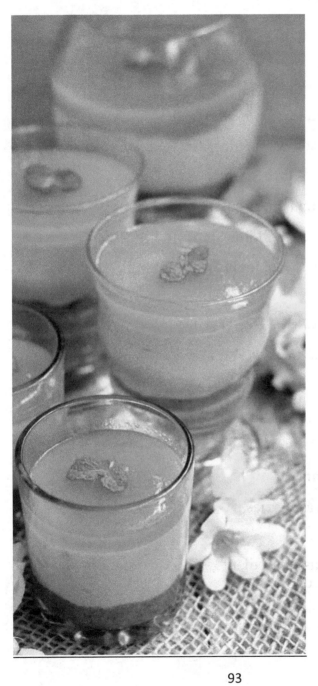

Cooking Time : 4 Hour 30 Minutes

Servings : 8 Servings

Ingredients:

Filling:

- 2 cups of Brazil Nuts
- 5 to 6 Dates
- 1 tablespoon of Sea Moss Gel (check information)
- 1/4 cup of Agave Syrup
- 1/4 teaspoon of Pure Sea Salt
- 2 tablespoons of Lime Juice
- 1 1/2 cups of Homemade Walnut Milk (see recipe)*

Crust:

- 1 1/2 cups of quartered Dates
- 1/4 cup of Agave Syrup
- 1 1/2 cups of Coconut Flakes
- 1/4 teaspoon of Pure Sea Salt

Toppings:

- Sliced Mango
- Sliced Strawberries

Directions :

1. Put all crust Ingredients, in a food processor and blend for 30 seconds.

2. With parchment paper, cover a baking form and spread out the blended crust Ingredients.

3. Put sliced Mango across the crust and freeze for 10 minutes.

4. Mix all filling Ingredients, using a blender until it becomes smooth

5. Pour the filling above the crust, cover with foil or parchment paper and let it stand for about 3 to 4 hours in the refrigerator.

6. Take out from the baking form and garnish with toppings.

7. Serve and enjoy your Mango Nut Cheesecake!

Blackberry Jam

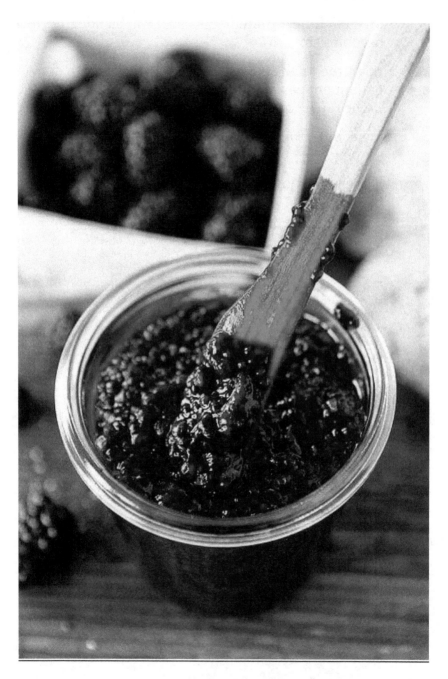

Preparation Time : 5 minutes

Cooking Time : 4 Hour 30 Minutes

Servings : 1 Cup

Ingredients :

- 3/4 cup of Blackberries
- 1 tablespoon of Key Lime Juice
- 3 tablespoons of Agave Syrup
- ¼ cup of Sea Moss Gel + extra 2 tablespoons (check information)

Directions :

1. Put rinsed Blackberries into a medium pot and cook on medium heat.

2. Stir Blackberries until liquid appears.

3. Once berries soften, use your immersion blender to chop up any large pieces. If you don't have a blender, put the mixture in a food processor, mix it well, then return to the pot.

4. Add Sea Moss Gel, Key Lime Juice and Agave Syrup to the blended mixture. Boil on medium heat and stir well until it becomes thick.

5. Remove from the heat and leave it to cool for 10 minutes.

6. Serve it with bread pieces or the Flatbread (see recipe).

7. Enjoy your Blackberry Jam!

Nutrition : Calories: 43; Fat: 0.5 g; Carbohydrates: 13 g

Blackberry Bars

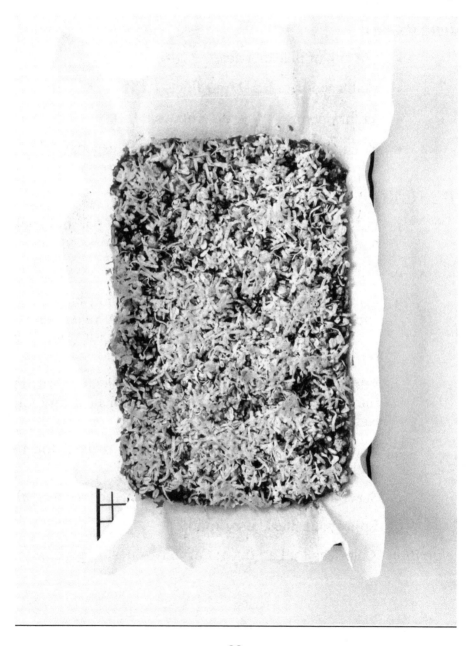

Preparation Time : 5 minutes

Cooking Time : 1 Hour 20 Minutes

Servings : 4

Ingredients :

- 3 Burro Bananas or 4 Baby Bananas
- 1 cup of Spelt Flour
- 2 cups of Quinoa Flakes
- 1/4 cup of Agave Syrup
- 1/4 teaspoon of Pure Sea Salt
- 1/2 cup of Grape Seed Oil
- 1 cup of prepared Blackberry Jam

Directions :

1. Preheat your oven to 350 degrees Fahrenheit.
2. Remove skin of Bananas and mash with a fork in a large bowl.
3. Combine Agave Syrup and Grape Seed Oil with the Blend and mix well.
4. Add Spelt Flour and Quinoa Flakes. Knead the dough until it becomes sticky to your fingers.
5. Cover a 9x9-inch baking pan with parchment paper.
6. Take 2/3 of the dough and smooth it out over the parchment pan with your fingers.
7. Spread Blackberry Jam over the dough.
8. Crumble the remainder dough and sprinkle on the top.
9. Bake for 20 minutes.

10. Remove from the oven and let it cool for at 10 to 15 minutes.

11. Cut into small pieces.

12. Serve and enjoy your Blackberry Bars!

Nutrition : Calories: 43; Fat: 0.5 g; Carbohydrates: 10 g; Protein: 1.4 g; Fiber: 5 g

Detox Berry Smoothie

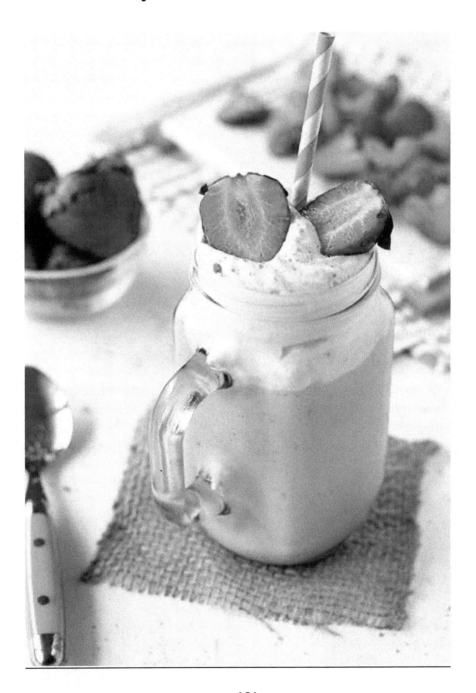

Preparation Time : 15 minutes

Cooking Time : 0

Servings : 1

Ingredients :

- Spring water
- 1/4 avocado, pitted
- One medium burro banana
- One Seville orange
- Two cups of fresh lettuce
- One tablespoon of hemp seeds
- One cup of berries (blueberries or an aggregate of blueberries, strawberries, and raspberries)

Directions :

1. Add the spring water to your blender.
2. Put the fruits and vegies right inside the blender.
3. *Blend all Ingredients till smooth.*

Nutrition : Calories: 202.4; Fat: 4.5g ; Carbohydrates: 32.9g ; Protein: 13.3g

Shredded Chicken Salad

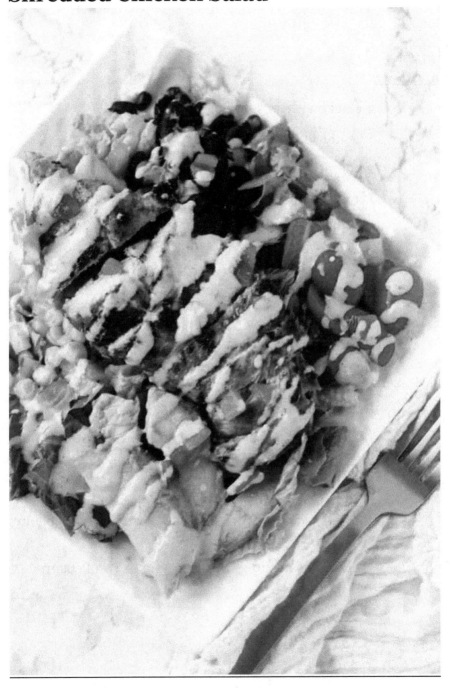

Preparation Time : 5 minutes

Cooking Time : 10 minutes

Servings : 6

Ingredients :

- 2 chicken breasts, boneless, skinless
- 1 head iceberg lettuce, cut into strips
- 2 bell peppers, cut into strips
- 1 fresh cucumber, quartered, sliced
- 3 scallions, sliced
- 2 tbsp. chopped peanuts
- 1 tbsp. peanut vinaigrette
- Salt to taste
- 1 cup water

Directions :

1. In a skillet simmer one cup of salted water.

2. Add the chicken breasts, cover and cook on low for 5 minutes. Remove the cover. Then remove the chicken from the skillet and shred with a fork.

3. In a salad bowl mix the vegetables with the cooled chicken, season with salt and sprinkle with peanut vinaigrette and chopped peanuts.

Nutrition : Carbohydrates: 9 g; Protein: 11.6 g; Total sugars: 4.2 g; Calories: 117

Broccoli Salad

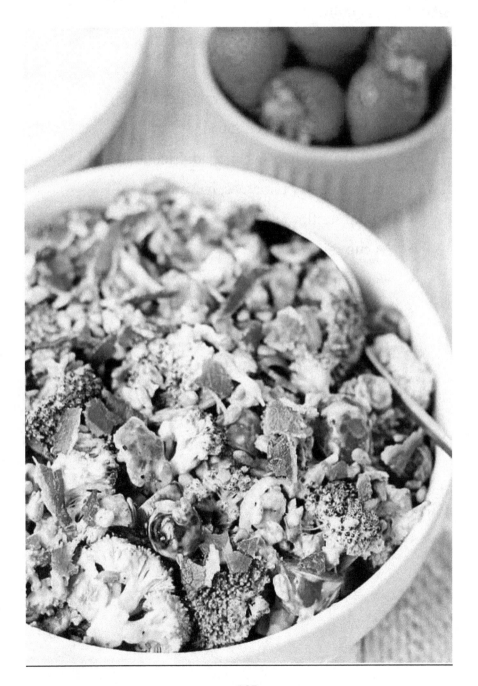

Preparation Time : 10 minutes

Cooking Time : none

Servings : 6

Ingredients :

- 1 medium head broccoli, raw, florets only
- 1/2 cup red onion, chopped
- 12 oz. turkey bacon, chopped, fried until crisp
- 1/2 cup cherry tomatoes, halved
- ¼ cup sunflower kernels
- ¾ cup raisins
- ¾ cup mayonnaise
- 2 tbsp. white vinegar

Directions :

1. In a salad bowl combine the broccoli, tomatoes and onion.
2. Mix mayo with vinegar and sprinkle over the broccoli.
3. Add the sunflower kernels, raisins and bacon and toss well.

Nutrition : Carbohydrates: 17.3 g; Protein: 11 g; Total sugars: 10 g; Calories: 220

Cherry Tomato Salad

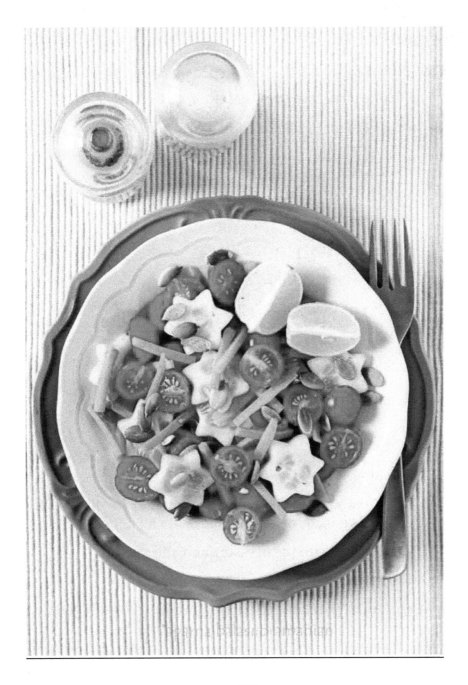

Preparation Time : 10 minutes

Cooking Time : none

Servings : 6

Ingredients :

- 40 cherry tomatoes, halved
- 1 cup mozzarella balls, halved
- 1 cup green olives, sliced
- 1 can (6 oz.) black olives, sliced
- 2 green onions, chopped
- 3 oz. roasted pine nuts

Dressing:

- 1/2 cup olive oil
- 2 tbsp. red wine vinegar
- 1 tsp. dried oregano
- Salt and pepper to taste

Directions :

1. In a salad bowl, combine the tomatoes, olives and onions.
2. Prepare the dressing by combining olive oil with red wine vinegar, dried oregano, salt and pepper.
3. Sprinkle with the dressing and add the nuts.
4. Let marinate in the fridge for 1 hour.

Nutrition : Carbohydrates: 10.7 g; Protein: 2.4 g; Total sugars: 3.6 g

CPSIA information can be obtained
at www.ICGtesting.com
Printed in the USA
LVHW080754110721
692393LV00002B/55